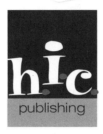

This book was made possible
in part by an unrestricted grant from
GENENTECH INC.

Hope Lives!

The After Breast Cancer Treatment

Survival Handbook

Compiled by Margit Esser Porter

h.i.c. publishing

P.O. Box 3026

Peterborough, N.H. 03458

P.O. Box 3026
Peterborough, N.H. 03458
Copyright © 2000 by Margit Esser Porter

Designed by J Porter & Doreen Abraham

Manufactured in the United States of America
5 7 9 10 8 6 4
Publisher Cataloging-in-Publication Data
Porter, Margit Esser.
Hope Lives!: the after breast cancer treatment survival handbook /
compiled by Margit Esser Porter.
192 p.   16 x 16 cm.
1. Breast—Cancer—Patients—Quotations.
2. Breast—Cancer—Patients—Attitudes. I. Title.
RC280.B8P665a—2000
362.1'9699449—dc21   00-104204
ISBN 0-9700443-0-5   CIP

Dedication

THE INTENT OF THIS BOOK is to help
those who are living with, and recovering from,
breast cancer treatment. It is not written by
doctors and is not intended to replace the advice
of medical caregivers or your own common sense.

Contents

❧

"If an Arctic summer

is exceptionally cold, some 'snow-bed' plants may not emerge

at all from underneath deep drifts. But they survive, biding

their time for another, more favourable year. . . . Buried in

a permafrost, they can survive millennia. A lemming's cache

of Arctic lupine seeds, hidden deep in the frozen ground

more than ten thousand years ago, was recently discovered by

botanists. Given earth and light and water, these seeds, asleep

for one hundred centuries, awoke to life; they germinated, grew

roots and flowers and new seeds. These delicate, lovely plants

were older than mankind's recorded history."

— FRED BRUEMMER, *Seasons of the Eskimo*

Hope Lives!

Foreword

I PAUSED RECENTLY, in front of one of the great university libraries, and wondered where all that knowledge, accumulated over centuries of effort, had gone, how much of it was empty of human purpose. This is a book about knowledge that helps. It is about women telling what they did and do to make their lives easier while grappling with breast cancer.

When Margit was diagnosed with breast cancer in 1995, she was by her own description "curled up in a fetal position." Underneath that fear and panic was something waiting to develop into the empowered woman who transforms her hellish experience into a wonderful handbook for her fellow travelers. Margit gleans the wisdom of hundreds of women with breast cancer. They tell how to soften the blow of the tense times that follow the diagnosis and give that invaluable perspective of experience. And who better to be your guide than those who have "been there, done that" and figured out a way to survive, even making things a little better and even letting you laugh a bit?

This book should be a powerful inspiration to its readers and keep oncologists humbled and in awe. From her position of helplessness, Margit grew into a courageous woman determined to help every other "curled-up fetus" out there.

❧

Margit incorporates all that she has learned to transform her own life. She then becomes the ultimate patient advocate in sharing her acquired wisdom. She is the embodiment of the power of the human spirit, and every reader will find her hope and inspiration contagious.

—ANNETTE FURST, M.D.
Oncologist, Faulkner Breast Centre, Boston

Introduction

I AM WHAT PEOPLE REFER TO as a "breast cancer survivor." The term is used to describe any person who is alive after diagnosis. Taken literally, I guess this means if hearing the diagnosis doesn't kill you, you're a survivor. The word "survivor" has always confused me. Perhaps I watched too much television as a child, but it bothered me that surviving the wreck of the SS MINNOW meant that Gilligan was left with nothing to do except wait day after day for rescue.

I also grew up in a family riddled with cancer. When my older sister died of it at the age of ten, and my mother at the age of forty-seven, I learned to think of a survivor as someone who DIDN'T get cancer. Wasn't I the one surviving a wreck and waiting for rescue? So it seems strange to me that it was only when I reached the age of thirty-four and was myself diagnosed with cancer, that people would begin to call me a survivor.

In an effort to make peace with a word that is now freely used to describe my relationship to a dreaded disease, I have created my own definition. In my mind, survival represents obtaining the skills and tools necessary to enjoy a decent quality of life regardless of the length of life. It is not merely about existing, but about living life fully. The tool I use and value most is hope!

Each year 185,000 women are diagnosed with breast cancer, and approximately 45,000 die of the disease. Several thousand others live with it for many years. When cancer treatment is completed, these women need support, encouragement, and sound advice on how to resume their lives. They need answers to questions regarding issues such as posttraumatic stress, body image, fear of recurrence, living with recurrence, physical limitations, discrimination, and self-esteem. Many of these questions can best be addressed by others in the same situation. I know about these needs from my own experience.

On Friday the thirteenth of October 1995, I was diagnosed with breast cancer. The superstitious would say that Friday the thirteenth is a day when such bad luck occurs. Indeed, it was the day that I found out I had cancer, but it was also the day I began to treat it and get well again.

While undergoing treatment, I circulated a questionnaire across the country, collecting advice, support, and wisdom from other women with breast cancer. Their responses served not only to get me through my treatment but also to become volume one of what I affectionately call a six-by-six-inch paperback support group. Others call it HOPE IS CONTAGIOUS: THE BREAST CANCER TREATMENT SURVIVAL HANDBOOK. Since the publication of HOPE IS CONTAGIOUS, I have met and spoken with thousands of women of all ages and with all stages of breast cancer. They share a strong desire to help others even while in the midst of their own crises. Every woman I talk with clearly remembers when she was first diagnosed, and each has some valuable advice or piece of wisdom to offer on getting through treatment and living life with breast cancer.

As I read the comments of these women, I realize that breast cancer has permanently changed their lives, just as it has permanently changed mine. I have no desire to go back to being the person I was before all this happened; my entire outlook on life is different now. This shift is not unique to me or even to women with breast cancer. It is characteristic of virtually anyone who faces a serious illness. That's part of the reason that the insights of these special women provide a valuable perspective on life after diagnosis and treatment not only for breast cancer survivors but for those dealing with other serious illnesses as well.

Hundreds of new voices make up this book, as well as a few familiar names from volume one. The familiar names are older now; these women have lived with breast cancer longer and are eager to share more advice. Many of them feel like old and trusted friends, and their continued presence in this new title is itself a reaffirmation that HOPE IS CONTAGIOUS and HOPE LIVES!

Breast wishes!

MARGIT ESSER PORTER

Chapter One

Family, Friends & Work

"I'm renewing a friendship with a woman I had

neglected for a very long time . . . ME!"

— TINA, *age 54, diagnosed 1998*

"I was diagnosed with breast cancer on Mother's
Day 1981 and have been living with metastatic
breast cancer and the absence of remission since.
What I thought and certainly felt, though briefly,
was my death sentence has become my greatest
strength and worthwhile challenge. First as a police
officer and now as a sergeant and commander of
the Domestic Violence Unit for the Boston Police
Department, I have seen what domestic violence does
to those who survive and the one too many who have
been murdered through the atrocities of violence. It
is the strength of these women, children, and men
that gives me the true power and inspiration to
NEVER GIVE UP. I reflect on the faces of those whose

spirit has been broken if not destroyed, and I remind myself of how lucky I am."

— *Sergeant Detective, Commander of the Domestic Violence Unit,*
Boston Police Department,
GLADYS AQUINO GAINES, *age 42, diagnosed 1981*

"When I was diagnosed with breast cancer, my mother had just died of ovarian cancer after having had breast cancer. My family was very supportive of me, but I could sense their fear. Now that treatment has ended, we make the most of each day, taking advantage of the here and now instead of wasting time planning and acquiring."

— TRICIA, *age 38, diagnosed 1998*

"I was afraid that people at work would always think of me as a weak and vulnerable person after having seen me sick for so long. I thought I'd lose my position on the corporate ladder when treatment ended. I was wrong. In fact, it was quite the opposite. They see me as being strong for having gotten through such a difficult ordeal."

— BARBARA, *age 46, diagnosed 1997*

"My husband couldn't accept that cancer had changed me. All he saw was that I was different, and he missed the old me. We split up. I thought the stress would surely cause a recurrence. The old me is gone, but the young new me now has a new young boyfriend."

— GRACE, *age 37, diagnosed 1994*

"I was diagnosed during my first year of marriage! I couldn't have made it through without my husband's support. I am still married to the same wonderful guy. Getting through diagnosis, treatment, and the aftermath together strengthened our marriage." — EVELYN, *age 53, diagnosed 1990*

"When treatment ended, I began thinking about dating again. One of the main questions I had was, would anyone want to get close to me once they knew I had cancer? My breast had some obvious scar tissue internally in one area. Should I tell someone I had cancer before we became physically involved? What I realize is that I need to take each person as an individual and check it out with myself as I get to know each man I date. I am also very aware of not wasting time with the wrong person."

— LISA, *age 43, diagnosed 1997*

"I started dating a nice man after my treatment ended, but I wouldn't have sex with him because I was afraid of being seen naked. By nature I'm a pessimist, and I was convinced he'd be put off by a woman with only one breast. Luckily, he was an optimist with a great sense of humor. He tried so many times to put the moves on me, and because I hadn't told him about my mastectomy, he couldn't understand what the problem was. As the months passed, he finally asked me at dinner one night why I wouldn't allow him to get closer. I told him that I had once had cancer and it had left me with some physical changes. The words 'breast cancer' were never expressed, just 'cancer.' He smiled and replied that he had had an injury back in college that had left him with an altered physique. When I asked him what he was talk-

ing about, he replied, 'Well, I guess you could say
that as a pessimist, you see yourself with a cup half
empty' (referring to my bra cup), 'and as an optimist,
I see myself with a cup half full' (referring to his athlet-
ic cup). Ever since that night, we've had great sex, and
we've been happily married for six years!"

— LEE, *age 52, diagnosed 1991*

"My husband is a survivor of the Vietnam War. We
were married for twenty-six years before I was diagnosed. Once I allowed him into my inner circle, he
was able to share his survival skills with me. Now
we have more respect for each other. We have a very
loving, strong, and better marriage."

— MARILYN, *age 47, diagnosed 1997*

"My relationships with friends have pretty much stayed the same as before I had cancer, except that now I know who will be there for me in a time of crisis and who will watch from a distance. That's not such a bad thing to find out at my age." — JO, *age 31, diagnosed 1996*

"My husband started seeing another woman while I was in the middle of treatment. Every time I tried confronting him about it, he would lie and tell me that my side-effect drugs were making me paranoid. I believed him because I was too scared not to. Both my treatment and his affair have ended. Hoping to prevent a recurrence of cancer and infidelity, we've added a marriage counselor to our list of specialists." — CAITLIN, *age 49, diagnosed 1998*

"My bad marriage got better while I was in treatment because I didn't have the time or energy to focus on anything else and because my husband felt too guilty to leave me or hurt me while I was down. After treatment ended, we both realized that I was going to live but our marriage had to die."

— SARAH, *age 31, diagnosed 1994*

"It has been five years since my treatment ended. I am still working as a bank teller in the same community. Working throughout my treatment not only kept me busy so I did not dwell on my bad luck, it also helped me realize how caring and supportive people can be."

— BARBARA, *age 54, diagnosed 1994*

"My private health insurance rates went way up after my treatment ended. I got really scared because I couldn't afford the increase and I knew I'd never be able to prove discrimination. The law would not allow the company to cancel my plan, but the rate hike was supposedly allowed. After calling a lawyer friend of mine, I found out that I could shop for a new insurance company and get the rates in writing without having to disclose any preexisting conditions. I ended up moving my health care to a better insurance company with a less expensive monthly premium. My advice is, don't wait until the eleventh hour. Shop now for the best insurance policy."

— SADIE, *age 40, diagnosed 1997*

"Because financially I could afford to, I stopped working while I was in chemo. Big mistake! Getting back into the job market after dropping out for so long is not easy to explain, and people aren't exactly eager to hire a potential-sick-day employee. I also found out that not working gave me too much time to think. Until I get a paying job, I'm doing volunteer work just to keep busy."

— JODY, *age 48, diagnosed 1997*

"I quit my job when I was diagnosed. Though I can't afford to stay unemployed forever, I am really enjoying this time for myself."

— JILLIAN, *age 29, diagnosed 1999*

"I'm a teacher, and the timing of my treatment was excellent because it started just as school was ending for summer break. I didn't have to worry about missing too much work. On the last day of school, about fifteen of my colleagues, along with my entire eighth-grade class of students, held a 'get well soon' party for me. They surprised me with gifts and an enormous cake. The best, and by far the funniest, gift they gave me was the fact that EVERYONE, faculty and students alike, had shaved their heads. They claimed we would ALL have our hair back for the new school year, and if not, then they'd shave again!"

— FRANCES, *age 45, diagnosed 1997*

"Work has always been the place where I get my strength. I worked throughout my treatment except for when I had to be in isolation in the hospital during my bone marrow transplant. I went back to work just as soon as possible when I got out of the hospital. I don't know how I'd cope if I didn't have this job. It gives me money, self-esteem, a focus, a feeling of security in a world gone wrong, and a place to go where I am respected and needed."

— SLOAN, *age 47, diagnosed 1998*

"The only thing more threatening to my well-being than the tumor was my inability to face it. I am dealing with it now. I feel liberated."

— BRENNA, *age 31, diagnosed 2000*

"I never worked until I had cancer. After my treatment ended, I wanted to give something back, so I started volunteering at my hospital helping newly diagnosed women cope with the trauma of breast cancer. I inspire people because I'm doing so well, and I'm doing so well because I inspire people."

— ANNETTE, *age 77, diagnosed 1988*

"I am much more religious now than I used to be."

— PAULA, *age 62, diagnosed 1996*

"When I see something I want now, I buy it. Before cancer, I was so cheap with myself."

— CAROLYN, *age 39, diagnosed 1999*

"No matter what, I take the time to exercise each day. I tell myself that this is no longer a time slot to give away. Now the phone goes unanswered, the E-mail gets ignored, or the laundry doesn't get folded. But every morning I get my walk, and I use the dog as an excuse when people try to steal that hour from me. I just say that I have to take the dog for a walk, and off we go for a long, long, long, walk."

— NOREEN, *age 44, diagnosed 1996*

"People think I'm healthy now so it's okay to dump on me again. They were so careful around me when I was in chemo. Why do I have to feel sick for people to treat me well? I think I need some new friends."

— KRISTIN, *age 41, diagnosed 1998*

"Some people have actually asked me why I can't just put this 'breast cancer thing' behind me and get on with my life. As if I won't be truly healed until I can abandon the subject. I want to tell these people that if I were an alcoholic and needed to go to AA meetings three times a week, they'd applaud my courage and my goal of sobriety. But this disease, this breast cancer, which was not self-inflicted, has its own serenity prayer. God grant me the serenity to tolerate idiots!"

— MARGIT, *age 39, diagnosed 1995*

"I value time more now, and it shows in little ways. I won't talk on the phone while I'm eating breakfast or late at night. When I'm put on hold, I hang up."

— HEIDI, *age 66, diagnosed 1999*

"I took a leave from work while I underwent treatment, but I never told anyone why. Now I'm back at work and no one is the wiser, but I feel as though I were raped and I never reported it."

— GAIL, *age 56, diagnosed 1996*

"It took me three years to work up the courage to walk around the locker room at my health club without covering up my scars with a towel. When I finally got up the guts to be naked, nobody even noticed. The steam room was too steamy, and most women were too busy covering up their own imperfections to notice mine."

— SHIRLEY, *age 43, diagnosed 1993*

"My partner is a woman, too, and unusually accepting of me and all of the changes cancer brought into our life, including our sex life. Because we are both female, I haven't had to explain the changes in my body. She has made it clear that I am still desirable to her, and as long as we don't rush things or expect them to be just the same as before cancer, we've kept the spark and connection between us very much alive." — LAURIE, *age 46, diagnosed 1998*

"My work life continues. I answer my phone to hear a patient/friend weeping: she is at her surgeon's office and has been told that her breast cancer has spread to her brain. I sit with a patient/friend whose initial presentation was very much like my own; she now has widely spread metastatic disease. I accompany a patient/friend to her initial consultation with the bone marrow transplant

team. I sit with a dying woman and her daughter, who is
exactly the same age as my younger girl; we talk and plan
together for the girl's life after her mother's death. My
brain and my heart are exploding. How can I possibly
help this woman when I am so overwhelmed by my own
fear and grief? How can I not when helping her means
helping me? It is the best way I can fight back."

— Chief Oncology Social Worker
for the Beth Israel Deaconess Medical Center, Boston
HESTER HILL SCHNIPPER, *age 50, diagnosed 1993*

"After treatment finished, I had a lot of depression
and fear. A support group at my local hospital helped
me a great deal. As more time goes by, I sometimes
find myself actually forgetting what I went through."

— SUSAN, age 58, diagnosed 1997

"I didn't join a support group until after my treatment for breast cancer was completed. Chemo was enough of a distraction, and it took most of my energy. I'd like to think I can put all of this behind me, but I just can't get beyond the fear. The support group helps me realize that I'm normal. When I see women who are years past treatment, I'm given hope that I too will work through this."

— ELLEN, *age 41, diagnosed 1995*

"I left my support group because too many of the women in it were in really bad shape and it depressed me. I use the time to treat myself to a massage each week and to meditate daily."

— EMILY, *age 57, diagnosed 1996*

"I made a lot of friends in my support group, and I didn't want to leave them just because I was done with treatment. I still go to the meetings, though not as much as before. We celebrate birthdays with fattening junk (those of us who are old-timers have all put on a few pounds), and those who haven't done well have taught me valuable lessons about accepting death when the time is right. My life is richer because of all of these women."

— LAURA, *age 63, diagnosed 1997*

"I made a really good friend when I was in treatment. We have both done well, and we continue to be friends to this day."

— MARIANNE, *age 36, diagnosed 1996*

"During my treatment, I maintained the attitude that you did what you had to do, there wasn't a choice. I believe this has something to do with why I hate it when people tell me how brave I was. Bravery is when you choose."

— BECKY, *age 32, diagnosed 1997*

"People often tell me how good I look, in the mistaken belief that they are paying me a compliment. I always want to reply by telling them that I looked great the day that I was diagnosed with breast cancer, but instead I just say thank you. It beats the alternative 'How are you feeling?' question that I get asked too often. Let's face it. There's no right question."

— JACQUELINE, *age 49, diagnosed 1996*

"Early on Thanksgiving morning, when I had just gotten out of bed, with my new head of hair sticking up in every direction, my brother, concerned for my well-being, told me that I looked awful. He, in his panicky and overprotective way, was worried that the cancer was back. It made me angry, so I told him that if breast cancer were judged on appearance, he'd be metastatic!"

— LESLIE, *age 34, diagnosed 1996*

"I feel much more spiritually rooted since treatment. This has been nurtured by my support group and others in my faith community."

— MAUREEN, *age 48, diagnosed 1993*

"I've always been very driven, and it was hard for me to learn to shut that off, because work was the only thing that I could control in my life. I still like to do a good job, but I no longer sweat the small stuff."

— TRICIA, *age 38, diagnosed 1998*

"I think I'm more tolerant of people. I recognize that almost everyone has a terrible problem (or two or more). Be it a health problem or an emotional problem or a relationship problem. No one scoots along in life untouched by some tragedy. So when I meet people or am in a group, I keep in mind that everyone is struggling with personal problems."

— EVELYN, *age 53, diagnosed 1990*

"Cancer treatment seems to have altered more than just my DNA. I have a different outlook on life. I've started doing things I've never done before, like eating meat after being a vegetarian for twenty-four years. I have zero tolerance for negativity or gossip. My hair has grown back thick and curly and darker. I've started playing hooky from work to go to Red Sox games and have taken up watching ESPN! My husband, loving all of these changes, has started calling me Loretta. He claims this fulfills his fantasies because he can feel as though he's having an affair with this totally different woman to whom he just happens to be married."

— MARGIT, *age 39, diagnosed 1995*

"I no longer fund my IRA; instead I use the money to go to Hawaii." — TRICIA, *age 38, diagnosed 1998*

"I have the same job, but I have tried to balance my needs better. I don't offer to do more than I am expected to do. I spend time now with family and friends and have some individual time to pursue my interests, such as quilting, reading, and exercising."

— MAUREEN, *age 48, diagnosed 1993*

"It has been four years since I was diagnosed and underwent treatment. My friends have had so many changes in their lives during that time. Some have gotten married; some have had children. They've switched jobs, been promoted, you name it. I feel like all I've done is go to war and come home again. It's hard to explain, but I feel like I've been in a time warp and I don't know how to relate to people the same way.

When people ask what I've been up to lately, thinking that cancer is long behind me, how do I reply? Do I say, 'Well, while you've been off making something of your life, I've been barely hanging on to mine'? Part of me just wants to move far away and start all over again. This has prompted me to take some time off from work and travel for a while."

— DELIA, *age 32, diagnosed 1996*

"Before I had cancer, much of my time and money were spent trying to look perfect. I still believe in vanity, but I'm no longer obsessed with my outward appearance. I realize now that my friends and family love me for more than my looks."

— MOLLY, *age 38, diagnosed 1993*

"I must admit I had some concerns about leaving my previous place of employment after treatment was over. They were a known to me. But . . . I deserve to be able to create a life that makes me happy. I did check out the health insurance plan before I committed to taking a new job and made sure that all of my doctors were covered participants in the plan. I knew what all the benefits were in advance of accepting the new position."

— LISA, *age 43, diagnosed 1997*

"I'm still married to a truly great man and husband. I recently asked him how he could still love me. I am such a different person than I was four years ago. He grinned and replied that he was banking on me changing!"

— SHARON, *age 36, diagnosed 1996*

"One of my close friends couldn't deal with my decision to have chemo, so she became angry and stopped speaking to me. I have forgiven her and moved on. It had little to do with me and more to do with her own fears."

— NANCY, *age 47, diagnosed 1993*

"My daughter seems to take me less for granted now. She is aware that neither of us will live forever, but, more important, she no longer looks to me to be a pillar of indestructible strength. I am also less controlling of her than before. I just can't work up the energy to get upset about little things. We are both grateful to have more time together."

— VIOLET, *age 41, diagnosed 1995*

"My daughter was only a year old when I was diagnosed, and I am hoping that by the time she is old enough to understand what breast cancer is, we will have a cure for it. I would hate for her to have to live with the kind of fear that I live with."

— HILLARY, *age 34, diagnosed 1994*

"I was worried about my rights for health insurance and discrimination issues if I quit my job to take time to travel and relax a bit. I called the Patient Advocate Foundation (see Resources, page 173) and got a great deal of helpful information."

— POLLY, *age 44, diagnosed 1996*

"All the relationships in my life have changed, because I have been changed significantly by the experience of being diagnosed and treated. I think that my own identity as an individual has been strengthened. My relationship with my extended family is much different. I am more separate. I think my parents and sibling respect my need to take care of myself. My own life is the priority. My husband and daughter are next. I don't have much extra energy beyond that."

— SHARON, *age 36, diagnosed 1996*

"Just when my treatment was ending, my husband and I got news that the adoption we'd been waiting for would become final. And so life begins again."

— CAROLYN, *age 39, diagnosed 1999*

"Breast cancer affects the entire family. There are foundations that address the issues families face. You are not alone. Contact the Northeast Health Care Quality Foundation (see Resources, page 173) and ask about the It's My Fight Too and Bells and Silence for Remembrance campaigns." — BELINDA, *age 46, diagnosed 1999*

"There is no reason to exclude men from our fight against breast cancer. They can be strong advocates in the battle to find a cure. They can support and help us through treatment. And men do get breast cancer (though it is rare). There is even an organization called The Men's Crusade Against Breast Cancer (see Resources, page 168)." — KIM, *age 48, diagnosed 1999*

"I believe that long after we are gone from this planet, our work continues in the presence of those who carry us in their memories. At any rally, walk, run, or fundraising event for breast cancer, you will see in the faces of the families and friends of women who have had the disease, a determination to raise awareness about breast cancer and the hope for a cure. For every husband, life partner, child, sibling, parent, and friend who raises his or her voice, there is the presence of a woman who can no longer speak. In an effort to eradicate breast cancer, those who speak out remind us that HOPE LIVES!"

— MARGIT, *age 39, diagnosed 1995*

Chapter Two

How Is
My Health?

"I try to slow my racing mind by writing in

my journal or taking a long walk."

—SHARON, *age 36, diagnosed 1996*

"There are a number of people in my life who have suggested that because I didn't die of breast cancer, my cancer must not have been as aggressive as the doctors told me it was. This kind of thinking makes me angry. Just because something doesn't kill you doesn't mean it isn't deadly. I'm not looking to be pitied, but I'm bothered by the ignorance that society has about those of us who have not been defeated by cancer and are still living with it every day. In this world of E-mail, fax machines, and computers that get faster and faster, it seems people expect quick answers and compact solutions: cancer to kill you or medicine to cure you. Breast cancer doesn't work that way. People need to know that."

— HILLARY, *age 34, diagnosed 1994*

"Weight gain, weight gain, weight gain! I'm trying to be accepting of and at peace with my new, rounder body. It's not easy. I am grateful for the gift of living as long as I have, of seeing my grandchildren; something my mother didn't have. As of my last birthday, I have now outlived both my mother (who had breast cancer) and my maternal grandmother. It's an amazing, humbling feeling."

— SUSAN, *age 57, diagnosed 1996*

"My doctors, especially one surgeon, are very surprised I'm doing as well as I am. I chalk it up to a positive attitude, being as active as possible, and having a focus (for me, our two young daughters to raise)."

— CINDY, *age 47, diagnosed 1993 & 1997*

"I used to obsess about my health, but now I don't anymore, because I believe if I was resilient enough to withstand breast cancer and all the chemo drugs, I can withstand just about anything. As crazy as this sounds, it took me getting REALLY sick to stop being afraid of illness."

— MONIQUE, *age 52, diagnosed 1999*

"I have a lot of joint pain (from chemo), but I'm working on exercising to get back in shape and build myself up again. I need to regain mobility in my shoulder, my arm, and my chest, so I exercise a little bit more each day."

— SUSAN, *age 53, diagnosed 1998*

"Since I finished treatment, I've had two bone scans, two chest x-rays, and several breast ultrasounds. Always I was physically fine but left feeling like a hypochondriac. Every pain, pimple, rash, or cough scared me that the cancer was back, so I would run off for testing. Finally, after almost three years of fear, I'm starting to relax. Now I wait a month to see if the pain goes away before I rush in for a scan or biopsy. If you're feeling like you'll always be afraid and never be able to relax again, think about me and what I just said. Have faith that time does help. It's almost like when someone dies. You never completely forget, but time makes the pain, sadness, and fear less immediate."

— ILEANA, *age 33, diagnosed 1997*

"I was extremely fatigued after treatment ended. It's hard to tell if it's just motherhood or the treatment that is causing my exhaustion. I've returned to work, but I work out of my home now instead of an office, so I no longer have to fight traffic. For the fatigue, I take naps, baths, and massages and get help caring for my children from family members."

— TRICIA, *age 38, diagnosed 1998*

"Exhaustion! I need lots of time to rejuvenate after I interface with the rest of the world. After putting energy toward others, I need to withdraw, rest, hide with my kitten under my blankets, do restorative yoga postures. I need quiet and solitude to balance."

— SHARON, *age 36, diagnosed 1996*

"Treatment ends, and no one tells you you're cured. Every time you have a sore lymph node or pulled muscle, there is always the question of metastasis. It's the stuff that keeps you up at night wondering what it will take to make you feel healthy again. For me it took getting rear-ended by a kid driving 60 miles an hour in a 25 mph zone. Miraculously, I walked away with only three broken ribs. The pain was far worse than that from any of my surgeries for breast cancer, but the fractures were all on the noncancer side. For the first time since my diagnosis, I actually had a doctor tell me that the bone pain I felt in my chest was definitely NOT CANCER. It was the first time I felt healthy in three years!"

— MARGIT, *age 39, diagnosed 1995*

"As tempting as it is to fall into the trap, try not to compare yourself to others when it comes to recovery from treatment. You'll save yourself a lot of anxiety. I remember thinking I'd have permanent alopecia because my hair didn't grow back as quickly as a friend's had after her treatment. My blood counts took longer to recover, too. But my hair did grow back, and my counts did eventually rebound. Watching and worrying didn't make it happen any faster."

— EDITH, *age 42, diagnosed 1996*

"I handled my diagnosis really well. I handled the treatment even better. It's the recovery that I'm not able to cope with. I can't relax. I keep thinking that since I was the one to find my cancer, I can't rely on doctors to stay on top of my health care. As with many other young women, my original tumor didn't show up on a mammogram. I'm told that the tumor marker tests are not reliable, so when they come back okay, I'm not comforted much. I feel like I'll never feel safe again. The only good that comes from all this anxiety is that I can honestly say I live each day as if it were my very last and have not wasted one moment of my life since my treatment ended." — SARAH, *age 31, diagnosed 1994*

"For my head, I have a breast ultrasound every four months, along with my annual breast MRI and mammogram. At this rate, my radiologist sees my breasts more than my husband, but hey, whatever works."

— MARGIT, *age 39, diagnosed 1995*

"Next year will be five years for me. I know there's no magic number and cancer can return at any time, but I'm less afraid than I used to be. It helps not having to go for testing so often. I'm only reminded once a year that I had cancer (when I go for my annual mammogram), and I always bring a friend with me."

— RONNIE, *age 42, diagnosed 1996*

"I have this silly routine that I do every year after I get good mammogram results. I go to a sexy lingerie store and buy new bras (shopping has always been how I relieve anxiety). I can't think of a better way to celebrate getting to keep my breasts for another year. I know it's ridiculous, but it's really lots of fun."

— PATRICIA, *age 39, diagnosed 1996*

"I didn't wear a bra for years after treatment. My old bras didn't fit right, and I was afraid that buying a new one would be a jinx or something. Finally, one Valentine's Day, my boyfriend gave me roses and a gift certificate to go buy new bras. With it was a note that said, 'Roses are red, violets are blue, you've bounced back from treatment, and I'm proud of you. Not to complain, but it's time to restrain, an ounce of that bounce—go buy bras that are new!' I laughed and took the hint."

— KAREN, *age 29, diagnosed 1997*

"Every time I look in the mirror, I am reminded by my missing breast that I had cancer. I'm thinking about having reconstruction so that at least in clothes I'll look more like my old self. I hate my prosthesis. It's time."

— SHARON, *age 48, diagnosed 1993*

"I couldn't stand the anxiety of still having one breast left that could get cancer. Rather than just rely on the Tamoxifen, I had my remaining breast removed. At least now I'm not lopsided, and I don't have so much anxiety. I know I can still have a systemic recurrence and I can still get breast cancer in the remaining tissue. But I'm happier not having breasts."

— LOIS, *age 56, diagnosed 1995 & 1997*

"Every time I complained of a problem that seemed to be a side effect of treatment, my oncologist would say it was because of radiation and my radiation oncologist would tell me it was caused by chemo. Nobody would tell me what to do to feel better. It took two years, but most of the problems I had resolved in time. The only thing that hasn't gotten better is the lymphedema, so I contacted the National Lymphedema Network (see Resources, page 172) and got a great deal of helpful information about coping with lymphedema."

— BOBBY, *age 59, diagnosed 1996*

"My hair grew back, and I just can't bring myself to cut it. It's way below my waist now!"

— EDITH, *age 42, diagnosed 1996*

"Depending on your health insurance policy, certain follow-up procedures such as breast MRI may require precertification. Without it, you could be required to pay the full cost of the procedure. Don't assume that your doctor's office will automatically take care of this for you. It's a good idea to contact both your doctor and your insurance company with the necessary information BEFORE your appointment date for authorization. In other words, help your doctor to help you."

— MARGIT, *age 39, diagnosed 1995*

"Weight gain? The only time in my life that I ever felt thin enough was when I was in the middle of chemo. If that's what it takes to feel thin, no thank you! I'd rather go for health and pleasure. I feel so different about my body. My scars and pains are constant reminders. My body is not the same. I am not the same."

— SHARON, *age 36, diagnosed 1996*

"After I underwent a bone marrow transplant for stage three inflammatory breast cancer, my periods stopped. I was at a loss over what to do with the one-hundred-piece economy pack of menstrual pads that I had purchased before treatment. I decided to stick them on my feet and skate around my hardwood floors collecting all the dust that had accumulated while I was in the hospital."

— CYNTHIA, *age 37, diagnosed 1999*

"I feel strongly that the sense of ourselves as sexual beings can be a path to healing and want The Breast Cancer Fund (see Resources, page 164) to facilitate an understanding of this new context for wellness. Women, in particular, understand the connection between the sacred and our sexuality and will be the ones to lead both sexes into the conversation.

"I was thrown into menopause after my first chemotherapy at the age of forty-two. Along with my hair and my breast, I lost my libido. Eleven years into menopause, I have minus levels of sexual hormones but have found a way to have a passionate sex life without chemicals or creams. If I can do it, anyone can."

— *Founder and Executive Director of The Breast Cancer Fund,*
ANDREA R. MARTIN, *age 54, diagnosed 1989 & 1991*

"When I was diagnosed with breast cancer, I found out at the same time that I was pregnant. I was told to abort the pregnancy and that if I didn't abort, I shouldn't be treated until after I delivered the baby. I had to consider both my life and the life growing inside me. Another doctor told me that I had a 50 percent chance of entering into early menopause with treatment and that I could be treated while I was pregnant (certain chemotherapy drugs don't affect the fetus). I was told that chemotherapy would not work for me if I waited until after I delivered. I chose to maintain the pregnancy while being treated. I now have a healthy daughter, and life goes on. Always listen to yourself; doctors don't know it all. You have to be your own advocate."

— BECKY, *age 32, diagnosed 1997*

"Menopause? I look in amazement at young people
now, as if they are another order of being, so vibrant,
beautiful, and alive. There's a great divide between us,
and I'm suddenly old, white-haired, and physically very
limited. Hot flashes, no sex drive, and very dry skin
with scars where I once had breasts. Sometimes I feel
a lot of grief, but mostly I'm overcome by the strange-
ness of it all. I let the fact that everything has changed
so fast blow me open to other possibilities. Every relationship, my sexual identity, my spirituality and cre-
ativity—everything is called into question, has to be
renegotiated, relearned. With the chance that I will get
it right this time, since I have nothing to lose and
since nothing scares me much anymore. Honesty, com-
passion, and love are winning out over fear and defen-

siveness. I feel very blessed most of the time for the opportunity to grow in these ways."

— DESIREE, *age 40, diagnosed 1996 & 1997*

"Sexuality and sex can definitely be a problem after breast cancer. I went into menopause, and while my sex drive was still there, the moisture, hormones, and spontaneity were going, going, gone. It was hard to accept this new me. I felt prematurely old. What helped pull me through the worst part of the adjustment was giving myself time to grieve all the changes and figure out what I wanted...then communicating that to my partner instead of expecting her to be a mind reader. This meant letting go of huge expectations about sex."

— LAURIE, *age 46, diagnosed 1998*

"I've decided that instead of menopause aging me, it has made me younger. Think about it....The last time my body had the freedom from the stresses of monthly menstruation, I was only ten years of age! I had energy, vitality, and my entire future ahead of me. Menopause is a physical change, and not just a state of mind, but I believe that if my mind recalls the blueprint of my youth, my body will follow."

— MARGIT, *age 39, diagnosed 1995*

"One year after treatment ended, I had to go into the hospital for minor knee surgery. I still had side-effect issues from my past breast surgeries and chemo. My blood counts were still low, and my left arm needed protection from the invasion of needles and blood pressure readings. And then there was the mental component of being back in the hospital. To aid my blood, I ate lots of blood-building fruits, vegetables, red meat, and immune herbal teas. I wore a 'lymphedema alert' hospital bracelet (see Resources, page 172) on my left arm, and I had the surgery in a different hospital than where I had had my chemo, so the environment was different. The surgery went well with no complications. It IS possible to have a history of breast cancer and still have an uncomplicated hospital stay. The key word is 'history.'"

— SALLY, *age 61, diagnosed 1997*

"The only pain I have is muscle stiffness. Yoga helps."

— SUSAN, *age 57, diagnosed 1996*

"My doctor prescribed antidepressants for my depression, which he said was caused by the early onset of menopause. I never took the drugs. I was tired of putting pills into my body. I knew well that my depression was caused by the early onset of thirty-five unwanted pounds. I hated the way I looked. My clothes didn't fit. My reflection in the mirror was a person I didn't want to be. Even though I was healthy and felt I should be grateful just for being alive, I was very sad about the way I looked. It was really hard work. Really hard. But with diet and exercise and time, I lost the weight and the depression without the aid of drugs. It's much harder to lose weight when you're in menopause, and you have a slower metabolism, but it can be done."

— INGRID, *age 37, diagnosed 1997*

"For menopausal systems, I find that exercise works the best. Without at least 30 minutes of daily aerobic exercise, I can't sleep. When I run or go for a good fast walk, I sleep through the night without night sweats."

— MELINDA, *age 41, diagnosed 1997*

"If you want to consume more soy in your diet but you can't stand tofu, there's a great product in the refrigerator section of most health food stores called Silk by White Wave Inc. It comes in different flavors. I love the chocolate. I drink it straight and also freeze it to make frozen pops. It's yummy as hot chocolate, too! I love tofu, but Silk is a nice alternative as a treat. It may just be a placebo effect, but soy seems to help me handle menopause better." — MARGIT, *age 39, diagnosed 1995*

"We know about issues common to cancer survivors. The first and most important is 'Am I a survivor? Will I survive this?' We understand that everyone is living on borrowed time, but we live with that knowledge. It is not like 'Maybe I will be hit by a truck tomorrow.' It is intermittent, usually unexpected, paroxysms of feelings that can quite literally take your breath away. Sometimes the fear is like a wildcat on our backs, claws digging in.

"As months pass, I have become more comfortable in my skin. I again fit my clothes, run most mornings, and brush a full head of hair. I try to trust my body. Always there are parallel tracks of hope and planning inside me; each decision must be marked by a two-angle lens: the 'maybe I will live for years' view and the 'maybe I will die soon' one. Every goal, plan, thought, and relationship must be forced through a double filter.

"I am part of an astonishing collection of women. I am so proud of my sisters as we, alone and together, live with breast cancer. I give thanks for my companions on this journey.

"I have found courage. I have been given grace. I love my life." — HESTER, *age 50, diagnosed 1993*

"After my treatment ended, both of my dogs got cancer, so I became the caregiver to cancer patients. The lesson they taught me was that it's no easier being on the other side. In some ways it's worse."

— MARGIT, *age 39, diagnosed 1995*

Chapter Three

Recurrence

"This time I let others gather
information for me. I was too
overwhelmed to do it myself."

— CLAIRE, *age 49, diagnosed 1995 & 1999*

"Just after you've been rediagnosed is probably the hardest time to find the strength to shop for a new doctor. That is what I had to do, because when I had my recurrence, my oncologist told me I was going to die. He had a bad attitude, so I shopped around until I found a doctor who was willing to help me fight the disease. Some would say I was in denial. If that's true, I've been in denial for six healthy years!"

— CAROL, *age 52, diagnosed 1991 & 1993*

"When you've been diagnosed with terminal stage four breast cancer, it's hard to decide whether to try more chemo or risk destroying the quality of life you have left. First of all, make sure you have an oncologist who believes in you and can elicit the healer within you. You need to feel a partnership if you're going to be in a potentially very difficult treatment which may not have any benefits. Then ask yourself this: Am I the kind of person who will be kicking myself if I don't at least try another treatment? Even if it doesn't work, will I die satisfied that I tried? As soon as I answered yes, the agonizing debate was over, and I was less fearful of the side effects. I was lucky; Taxol is working for now, and the quality of my life is greatly improved."

— DESIREE, *age 40, diagnosed 1996 & 1997*

"When I had a recurrence, my doctor was on leave. Just as I had gotten a second opinion with my original diagnosis, I decided that my doctor's absence was a good excuse to try another hospital—perhaps one that didn't treat breast cancer exclusively but instead all types of cancer. I was hoping I might have more options for protocols to choose from. What I found out was that the breast center which had treated me originally gave me pretty much the same medical options but much more emotional support. My advice is, if you have breast cancer, have it treated at a hospital that has a breast center."

— SUE, *age 48, diagnosed 1997 & 1999*

"In the days when I had my mastectomy, hospitals didn't have breast centers. You went into surgery not knowing if you'd still have a breast when you woke up. Breast cancer didn't have the public attention that it has now. There are so many more choices for health care today. I have breast cancer in my other breast now, and I'm still not going to a breast center. I like my big hospital that treats a variety of illnesses. Every time I see someone worse off than me, I am reminded of how lucky I am. When I see people who should have died but haven't, when they have cancer much more aggressive than mine, or AIDS, I am inspired to keep fighting. I don't want to sit in a breast center with a bunch of women who feel bad about what they've lost. I just want to move on."

— KAY, *age 72, diagnosed 1968 & 1994*

"When a really close friend of mine was diagnosed with recurrence just after my treatment was finished, I completely lost all composure. Unable to separate the pain of my grief for her from the pain of fear for myself, I was at a loss as to how to help either of us. Then I learned the art of self-hypnosis. The use of this valuable tool saved my life and our friendship. Hypnosis has helped me to draw upon internal resources that I hadn't known existed."

— MARGIT, *age 39, diagnosed 1995*

"I like to make chemo days as fun as possible. My husband and I often play Scrabble during treatments, and we've developed special 'chemo rules,' which basically give me free rein to cheat like crazy. During play, I like to have a drink. My treatment center serves wine on request, but that has always seemed far too refined. Instead, I've brought my own pint glass and a can of Guinness to sip on. I've also gone to chemo dressed as Elvira, with a long black wig, a black leather miniskirt, a fake nose diamond, flashing red-light earrings, and a matching red-feathered boa. This was, of course, for Halloween. For some reason, drinking that foaming glass of stout, cheating with impunity at Scrabble, and dressing eccentrically make me feel like a rebellious teenager, which, after almost five years of chemo treatments at various times during my life, helps me survive and thrive."

— *1988 Olympic Gold Medalist, Disabled Giant Slalom,*
DIANA GOLDEN BROSNIHAN, *age 37,*
diagnosed 1975, 1993 & 1996

"My first response to what they wanted to do (technically referred to as a chest wall resection) when my breast cancer reappeared was: OVER MY DEAD BODY! They were talking of cutting out ribs and goodness knows what else. I truly had trouble coming to a place of being able to agree, but I knew without it my chances were slimmer.

"I am here three years later, after that nightmarish time, to tell you that with very minor physical adaptations (because of three missing ribs, a major portion of my sternum gone, and everything between the ribs gone), I am very active physically and you couldn't tell what I've been through. I clear brush, garden, power-walk with friends, hike, swim, exercise on a ski machine, and keep up with two teenage daughters. The surgery and my attitude, diet, and physical activity have kept the cancer at bay. I may be pooped by 6:00 P.M., but I'm up by 5:30 A.M. and live an absolutely rewarding life. I rarely have to bow to my past treatments and surgeries. Was it worth it? A resounding YES!

"Trust your instincts. One oncologist told me I wouldn't live without a stem cell transplant. It just didn't feel right to me. So far, so good. Three years later, there is no gross metastasis, and that oncologist now agrees he was wrong. Trust yourself!"

— CINDY, *age 47, diagnosed 1993 & 1997*

"While I've had no recurrence, the fear of it never leaves me completely."

— RUTH, *age 78, diagnosed 1984*

"It's not easy to put my feelings on paper about the time that my daughter had a recurrence. Prior to the final diagnosis, there is a time of great concern and worry—afraid of that final word—and some denial.

"Then comes the word, and it's as if suddenly someone has hollowed out your insides. It's a sinking feeling, finding yourself at the bottom of a black pit. Then you are aware of who this involves and how positive and brave she is. You know there IS hope, and you begin to climb out of that awful dark place and you go on, supporting, helping where possible as the need presents itself, and being positive in actions and spoken thoughts. Then comes a time when you don't look back. You DON'T even think 'What if?' You FEEL full of hope, and you truly smile again."

— RUTH, *age 71, diagnosed 1989*

"I have had breast cancer three times since 1972. I am a survivor thank God! I do not wish to dwell in the past. I am enjoying life and living fully now."

— ANN, *age 72, diagnosed 1972, 1991 & 1997*

"Why do I keep going through treatment when there is no permanent cure? I ask myself this every time. There are no options other than death, which to me is no option. It's not that I fear death. I really don't anymore. I just love life too much to quit. It's a race against time. Treatment buys me time until they come up with new drugs or new ways to treat this illness. I'm not quitting."

— ROBIN, *age 38, diagnosed 1996, 1998 & 1999*

"One of the hardest decisions I faced in the beginning of my second breast cancer was whether to have a bone marrow transplant. I had enough nodes positive (twelve) that I qualified to enter a protocol that was looking to learn if bone marrow transplants were helpful in multinode-positive breast cancer women. There were two arms to the study: one side got the transplant; the other had to agree to the kind of chemotherapy the study was mandating, and that wasn't CAF, which my oncologist first advised for me. I read a book, talked with people who'd had bone marrow transplants and some who hadn't, and finally decided not to choose it. I was afraid I would be (randomly) chosen for the 'wrong' chemo and then would feel like a loser. My doctors were very supportive when

I relayed my decision. For a year or so after treatment, I worried I might have chosen wrong, but I finally settled down and understood I'd done what I needed to do for myself, and so it was the right decision."

— PERRY, *age 58, diagnosed 1987 & 1995*

"At my age, it was hard to find a doctor to help me fight the disease. Most treated me as though I had had a long life and since death is inevitable, it might as well be from breast cancer. They told me that treating cancer in the elderly is difficult because we don't tolerate aggressive treatment very well. Doctors hate to fail. I finally found a doctor who believed that the only failure would be in not trying to help me fight to live."

— PRISCILLA, *age 84, diagnosed 1982, 1990 & 1999*

"When I had my recurrence, I blamed my doctor. He had treated me and the treatment didn't work, so it had to be his fault. Then I blamed myself because I hadn't done all the things I told myself I'd do if I got better. Then I blamed my husband because he wasn't as strong as I wanted him to be. I blamed my children because they took my energy away by having needs that children have. I blamed my job because it took all the rest of my energy. I blamed God and the dog and every friend I had. And when I was all alone with no one left to blame, I finally directed my anger at the real culprit. I blamed the cancer and signed up for treatment. If you want to win a war, it helps to know who the real enemy is. Mine is breast cancer."

— JULIE, *age 45, diagnosed 1998 & 1999*

"The first three times, I chose chemo and traditional treatment, but it gets harder on my body and my head to keep going back into it. This time, I'm going to try some alternative approaches to cancer. My friends think it's because I'm giving up and want to die now. I wish they could understand that the treatment is unbearable for me, and with so few choices left, I'm choosing a different approach because I want to live now. Not just survive, but live."

— DEBRA, *age 43, diagnosed 1991, 1994, 1998 & 1999*

"If your hospital doesn't offer the protocol you want, find another hospital. This isn't a car you're buying; it's your life."

— WENDY, *age 44, diagnosed 1997 & 1999*

"E-mail is a wonderful way to communicate with friends and family when it comes to subjects like recurrence. I get tired of having to repeat the same depressing information over and over again. With E-mail, I just write it once and copy the people on my address list who want to be informed. This way, I don't tire myself out. I can also respond to E-mail based on my energy level and mood at the time. When I'm feeling very alone and I want the company of others I go on-line. Other days, I don't want to be intruded upon, so I keep the computer turned off. There's a lot of information on the Internet about breast cancer. Some days I read it. Some days I press the delete button. Doing this gives me a great sense of control."

— BETSY, *age 54, diagnosed 1995 & 1999*

"The first time I had breast cancer, my doctors said
I didn't need a Hickman, even though other people
I knew had them. Now my veins are shot, and I have
to have one. I wish I had insisted on one years ago, but
I was too insecure to challenge my doctors. I'm so grateful to have one now. It's much less traumatic to have
chemo infused and get blood drawn. I love my Hickman."

— CLAIRE, *age 49, diagnosed 1995 & 1999*

"I got lucky. Both times, my breast cancer has been in my
breasts. My nodes have been clean, and as far as we know,
it hasn't spread anyplace else. Basically, I've just gone down
a cup size in each breast. It's what I jokingly refer to as my
mandatory (as opposed to cosmetic) breast reduction."

— SANDY, *age 50, diagnosed 1995 & 1999*

"Sometimes I ask myself how I would go about a certain task if I had just received the news that I had a recurrence. Often that helps me prioritize better—cut to the quick, if you will."

— EVELYN, *age 53, diagnosed 1990*

"I've learned to talk about death, to read about it, even to sit with those who may be closer to it than I. That way, I'm becoming accustomed to the idea that we are all going to die, and that makes it easier to live today, it really does.

"We're all terminal, only we know it and noncancer people might not. Our job is to ignore the statistics and live today, to be where we are without constantly worrying about tomorrow. With my second breast cancer diagnosis five years ago, I had twelve nodes positive. My surgeon told me not to look at statistics. That was good advice. As one of the women in my book says, 'It's a crap shoot. I've known women who have died who shouldn't and I've known women who didn't die who should have.' I think people like me because I'm still alive. That's hope for you."

— *Speaker, Editor, Author of* LIVING WITH BREAST CANCER,
PERRY COLMORE, *age 58, diagnosed 1987 & 1995*

"I was allergic to Taxol, so they couldn't give it to me. I was scared that they wouldn't be able to treat me with anything else. But they did, and I'm fine now."

— MARY, *age 45, diagnosed 1995 & 1998*

"For the first year after my first surgery, I found it difficult to deal with the fear of recurrence. I finally stopped worrying, and then I got a new primary. Although I've developed severe lymphedema in both arms, I continue to work selling real estate and do all the things I love to do (play bridge, read, do needlepoint, and travel). I am just so happy to be alive. I now live my life as if I never had cancer."

— MARYANNE, *age 74, diagnosed 1974 & 1987*

"The second time was much less frightening for me because I knew so much more about breast cancer. Knowledge is power, so get informed."

— JUNE, *age 60, diagnosed 1978 & 1998*

"There was so much fear! I did learn that a lot of it came from not knowing or understanding my condition. Ask questions. When I got all the information, I became less fearful. Then I just turned the rest over to God."

— KATHRYN, *age 46, diagnosed 1993 & 1996*

"The first time I had breast cancer, I beat it by not allowing it to change my life. The second time, I beat it by not allowing it to change my life. The third time, it changed my life, and I allowed it to. Maybe I'll beat it this time."

— JAN, *age 52, diagnosed 1985, 1989 & 1991*

"In 1987, at the age of forty-two, I was on top of the world. I had good friends, a good job, and an active lifestyle. Then the alien world of breast cancer came toppling down on me. I did what many women do— follow the six-month chemotherapy regime. Been there, done that, move on. In 1993, it reared its ugly head again. It had metastasized in both lungs and the liver. Now I looked at it differently. With the help of the American Cancer Society and Eastern Mountain Sports, I founded the Adventure Weekend (see Resources, page 161) in New England, a program for women of all ages and stages of breast cancer to come together and share a common bond. The weekend offers a chance to remember what happened but also to heal and move on by encountering emotional and physical challenges. Women participate in yoga, kayaking, and cross-country skiing and have the ability to talk freely and support each other. The last event of the weekend is a ropes course, where they challenge themselves on a variety of activities thirty-five feet in the air. Invariably, when they complete the course there is a smile on every face and they all say, 'If I can do this, I can do anything.' When I started the program, I was proud of what I had accomplished. Now, several sessions later, I am truly humbled every time we have a weekend."

— *Founder of the American Cancer Society Adventure Weekend*,
BETTY BORRY, *age 56, diagnosed 1987, 1993 & 1995*

"With my second diagnosis and treatment, I was thrown into menopause. Many of my questions about the changes I've experienced have been answered by the American Menopause Foundation Inc. (see Resources, page 162)."

— NANCY, *age 46, diagnosed 1995 & 1999*

"After I finished treatment, I went off to a retreat to go fly-fishing. It was a free program called Casting for Recovery (see Resources, page 166). I met great breast cancer survivors, ate wonderful food, and had a weekend of fun I will never forget."

— PAULA, *age 44, diagnosed 1995 & 1997*

"Four years ago, when I was diagnosed, my husband started going to a support group at our hospital, for family members. He made friends who help him now through this difficult time. I'm glad he has that support. It's one less thing for me to worry about."

— FRANCINE, *age 51, diagnosed 1996 & 1999*

"I've had both breast cancer and ovarian cancer. I have no breasts and no reproductive system, but I'm still very much alive and very much a woman. I am living proof that there is life after cancer treatment. Try to remember that you went through it so that you could live. Don't waste time being afraid. LIVE your life!"

— MARGARET, *age 51, diagnosed 1990 & 1997*

"When I had my recurrence, I chose to leave my support group and find one with women who didn't freak out over the idea that sometimes breast cancer comes back. I didn't want to scare newly diagnosed women, and most of the women in my group were not able to look at me without panicking. They would ask me what kind of treatment I had had or how many lymph nodes, and I just knew they were thinking that they were safe because I hadn't been treated properly the first time. I didn't have the heart to tell them otherwise. I joined a group that had women with similar situations to mine. It's easier on all of us. I get help, and I'm not treated like a goner."

— TAMMY, *age 48, diagnosed 1997 & 1999*

"Treatment is not as bad this time. My doctor has my side-effect medications adjusted well, and mentally I am not as overwhelmed as when I was originally diagnosed. I wish I had been in remission longer, but I'm happy that there are still drugs out there to treat me. I still work, play tennis, and take care of my children. Breast cancer for me is a chronic illness, but one I seem to be able to live with. I'm grateful for that, but I pray daily for a cure."

— RUTH, *age 49, diagnosed 1995 & 1999*

Chapter Four

Living with Breast Cancer

"Yoga! Just do it! It's going to take

me into the new millennium (3000)!"

—BETSY, *age 73, diagnosed 1982*

❧

"After I finished treatment, I couldn't get past the notion that chemotherapy, surgery, and radiation had hurt my immune system. They had, after all, left me with low blood counts, costochondritis, and lymphedema. Prior to my cancer diagnosis and the treatment that followed, I had always considered myself to be very healthy. I was a vegetarian who consumed no refined sugar or alcohol. I didn't smoke, had minimal body fat, and ran three miles a day. But at the age of thirty-four, I still got an aggressive breast cancer. It upset me that in order to treat it, my body had to take such a beating of toxic drugs.

"The reality is that my body survived those drugs and my immune system was damaged long before it was introduced to chemotherapy. Otherwise, cancer never

would have been allowed to grow in the first place!
Once I stopped blaming treatment for my new self,
I was able to realize that it was a new improved self, not
a weakened and vulnerable one. Yes, I have side effects
from treatment, but I needed to remind myself that one
of those side effects is remission. Posttreatment, and
living with a history of breast cancer hanging over
me, I still run every day, but now I also eat chocolate,
enjoy a good glass of wine now and then, and eat meat
(I crave the animal protein). A wonderful Chinese
herbalist provides me with herbs to make me stronger.
If I am lucky enough to stay in remission for a long
while, we will never know if it was because of the
Adriamycin, the reishi mushrooms, or the chocolate."

— MARGIT, *age 39, diagnosed 1995*

"One of my biggest gifts for standing up strong against
the trauma was given to me by my life partner. She
told me whenever I feel myself slipping into the pain,
I should say to myself, I have breast cancer; breast cancer doesn't have me!"

— LAURIE, *age 46, diagnosed 1998*

"I have several E-mail addresses. One is strictly for
communicating with people who have breast cancer.
On the days that I don't feel like dealing with the
subject, I don't open the mail sent to that address."

— CLAIRE, *age 49, diagnosed 1995 & 1999*

"I value the relationships I have BOTH with my Western doctors, who treated my breast cancer using conventional medicine, and with my Eastern doctor, who has helped me recover from Western treatment. Kind of a yin-yang thing."

— MARGIT, *age 39, diagnosed 1995*

"Chocolate! Ever since I finished treatment, I love eating chocolate. I used to feel guilty and think it was bad for me—refined sugar, cocoa butter, and all that. Well, cancer was really bad for me, so now I figure chocolate couldn't be any worse for my body than cancer was. I truly believe that if I eat chocolate without guilt, it may actually even cure cancer!"

— AMY, *age 44, diagnosed 1997*

"As I look back at photographs of myself nursing my two children, I cannot fathom how my breast, which brought the joy of nurturing my babies from my own body, could turn on me and threaten my life. I trust that medicine will find a way to buy me enough time to see my children through many more years. But even as I look to new discoveries to save my life, I do not believe we should have to choose whether our research dollars go for treatment, early detection, or prevention. All are equally important. Finding preventable causes is too late for those of us already diagnosed, but what about the future? We must find out whether society is polluting the environment in ways that will cause breast cancer in our daughters and their daughters. I care passionately about the search for cancer risks because I have metastatic breast cancer. We cannot ignore the environment in that search."

> — *Co-CEO and Cochairman of Solomont Bailis Ventures,*
> SUSAN S. BAILIS, *age 54, diagnosed 1992*

"Ever since my hair grew back, I have made a conscious decision to use only organic nonchemical shampoos and conditioners (see Resources, page 177). Since I have this great, totally new head of hair (new right from the roots), I've decided to take really good care of it. I may be missing a breast and overweight from menopause, but I don't have split ends!"

> — SUE, *age 49, diagnosed 1997*

"Although I was diagnosed five years ago and am no longer in treatment, I am still 'living with breast cancer,' although it gets easier each year. While no one would choose to get cancer, few of us make it through life without any problems, and most of the time I actually think I'm fortunate. My cancer was found early, I've lived fifteen years longer than my mother, and my children are grown and happily married. As a long-time volunteer for the American Cancer Society, I was fortunate to have a built-in support group at the time of my diagnosis and now try to offer that same support to other women who are going through that terrifying time of an abnormal test, breast cancer diagnosis, or treatment selection process. For me, the support of other survivors has been as important to restoring my mental health as the medical establishment has been to regaining my physical health."

— *National Board Member of the American Cancer Society,*
BARBARA KEENOY LESTAGE, *age 57, diagnosed 1995*

"I don't like to use chemical creams on my skin, but ever since treatment, when I'm outside for any length of time, I burn quickly if I don't wear sunscreen. I use a chemical-free sun care product made from organic ingredients that I'm not allergic to, called Sol Creme (see Resources, page 181)."

— MARGIT, *age 39, diagnosed 1995*

"Menopause has made my skin so dry that sometimes I get inflamed, puffy eyelids. Most skin creams make my eyes flare up worse. I have found that what works best is to place a warm, wet green-tea bag on each eye lid. I'm not certain if it's the green tea or just the warm compress of the tea bag, but each time I try it, the swelling goes down."

— CYNTHIA, *age 54, diagnosed 1998*

"Get a bone density test if you are in early menopause. Then you will have a baseline from which to measure your bone health in the future."

— CONSTANCE, *age 41, diagnosed 1997*

"A friend taught me a trick well worth sharing: drink plenty of water when you have to have blood taken. Your veins will pop up and be easier to find."

— MARGIT, *age 39, diagnosed 1995*

"Many hospitals and breast centers have networking programs where newly diagnosed patients are matched up with women who have completed treatment and had a similar diagnosis, history, age, etc. Find these programs and take advantage of the resources they offer. In most cases, both the patient and the sponsor find support in each other. This support can be very helpful for the woman in treatment as well as the woman in recovery."

— CASEY, *age 33, diagnosed 1998*

"After I underwent treatment, I completely cleaned up my diet. I saw a nutritionist and asked my health insurance to pay for a one-time visit so I could learn about how to eat right. I'm not doing it just to avoid getting cancer again. I know that eating pizza, fries, and burgers didn't cause my cancer, but I want to be more respectful of my body. I don't take my health for granted anymore."

— JORDI, *age 27, diagnosed 1999*

"I still take an afternoon nap—a leftover habit from treatment that I thoroughly enjoy and refuse to give up!"

— FAY, *age 54, diagnosed 1998*

"When I travel on an airplane, I wear a compression sleeve on my arm to help control lymphedema on the side where I had the mastectomy. Try it. It really helps!"

— LAURA, *age 57, diagnosed 1992*

"I wear a product called The Original Bug Shirt (see Resources, page 181) when I know I'm going to be outdoors during mosquito or black fly season (which in New Hampshire is pretty much most any day that's not winter). This shirt is wonderful because it's made of a soft, lightweight, breathable material that protects me not only from bug bites but sunburn as well. If you want help guarding against lymphedema, this shirt is a good alternative to chemical repellents."

— MARGIT, *age 39, diagnosed 1995*

"One of the things I started treating myself to when I was in chemo was a weekly massage. It was a wonderful pampering gift that I gave myself. At the time, I couldn't afford it, but I didn't think I was going to live very long, so I decided it was a good way to use my money. I'm long past treatment, and I still can't afford the luxury of massages, but I've managed to keep up the routine—only it's monthly instead of weekly. I forfeit other extravagances for my monthly massage, and it's worth it!"

— DARCEY, *age 52, diagnosed 1995*

"I have found that swimming helps my lymphedema."

— MARGIT, *age 39, diagnosed 1995*

"I still see my psychiatrist. She understands what
I've been through, and I can tell her things that friends
don't want to hear. She lets me recover at the pace
I need to. She helps me cope with the fear."

— PENNY, *age 40, diagnosed 1997*

"I still have my port-a-cath. I don't like having to
have it flushed, but the maintenance of it is minor
compared to trying to find my veins. When a medical
person says that they can't draw from it, I hold out
for someone who will."

— LIANE, *age 43, diagnosed 1997*

"There are so many public reasons to become an activist for breast cancer, but mine is privately motivated. When I had my bone marrow transplant, all of my friends supported me and constantly checked up on my status. After treatment was over, most of them treated me as if I were cured. In general, that was good because I wanted to put the whole ordeal behind me, but part of me just couldn't let go. That part participates just once a year in a local Race for the Cure (see Resources, page 167). When I am surrounded by hundreds of men and women fighting breast cancer, I feel like I am involved in something bigger than myself. When I raise money from pledges that friends donate to the Susan G. Komen Foundation in my name, I feel supported and optimistic about my future."

— ANGIE, *age 37, diagnosed 1996*

"To help prevent infection on the side where I had surgery, I keep travel-size Neosporin antibiotic ointment in my purse in case I cut my hand or arm. I also keep a prescription for antibiotics in my wallet."

— MARGIT, *age 39, diagnosed 1995*

"Breast cancer taught me that I am going to die one day—maybe not of breast cancer, but certainly of something. So how do I want to live? That's the question. And the closest I've come to an answer in the fourteen years since my breast cancer diagnosis is that I want to live in an ongoing exploration of love and intimacy. That's what's important now."

— *Actor, Breast Cancer Activist,*
JILL EIKENBERRY, *age 52, diagnosed 1986*

Chapter Five

Happiness Is

"What makes me happy? Giving
hope to newly diagnosed women
by telling them I've been
free of cancer for twenty years."

— LAUREL, *age 73, diagnosed 1980*

"I try to experience happiness in the moment. Even in periods of great sadness or fear, I look for any measure of happiness I can find. I'm convinced it strengthens my immune system."

— MARGIT, *age 39, diagnosed 1995*

"Being able to get out and work makes me happy."

— MAXINE, *age 62, diagnosed 1997*

"Traveling makes me happy. Especially traveling to warm climates. I love being by the ocean."

— ELLEN, *age 35, diagnosed 1997*

"Bringing my kids home from college and watching them go back in the fall. Having the opportunity to watch my children grow puts a smile on my face and laughter in my heart."

— SHERRY, *age 45, diagnosed 1998*

"What makes me happy? Small things, I guess. My perennials surviving the winter, a clean car, seeing my mom smile, a phone call from my son, progress on our plumbing job at our new house (which we still don't live in), waking up in the morning."

— CHRISTINE, *age 45, diagnosed 1997*

"Happiness for me is finding out that there is pleasurable sex after menopause. Yes, ladies, it is possible! It took a year to get back my libido, but it returned. I thought sex was gone for good, but it came back! Don't stop trying, and don't give up hope."

— CHLOE, *age 50, diagnosed 1997*

"Happiness is treating myself to working out with a personal trainer twice a week and knowing in my heart that I deserve to do this for myself."

— TYLER, *age 40, diagnosed 2000*

"I'm enjoying cooking lessons and preparing healthier meals for my family."   — CARY, *age 42, diagnosed 1998*

"Happiness is finally accepting my body as beautiful by letting go of expectations about thin women and big breasts. Our society has made up rules about what our appearance should be. I've finally found joy in making my own rules and sticking to them. I've had so much radiation that I'm positively radiant. My beauty is not just skin deep."

— AMBER, *age 42, diagnosed 1995, 1997 & 1998*

"I've signed up to do a sixty-mile walk (see Resources, page 169) for breast cancer!"

— HARRIET, *age 70, diagnosed 1999*

"Happiness is not allowing my treatment to take over my life. It keeps me alive, but after almost five years of constant treatment, I am finally learning that I can live with this illness with only an occasional bad day and not have treatment impact my daily pleasures of walking, reading, working, and playing the piano."

— JEANNE, *age 40, diagnosed 1995*

"I won two lotteries—the one in eight that gave me breast cancer and the state lottery scratch ticket that I bought on the day I finished treatment. I'm the luckiest unlucky person I know."

— MAURA, *age 38, diagnosed 1999*

"Happiness is sitting in a warm sunny spot in my living room on my meditation cushion and meditating for half an hour every morning."

— ALICIA, *age 52, diagnosed 2000*

"Every year my hospital throws a gala auction fundraising event for the Breast Centre. I attend because I get great pleasure being with people who raise thousands of dollars to support the place that saved my life. I love seeing my doctors all dressed up in gowns and tuxedos, dancing and smiling and not talking shop (even though they're all wearing beepers). When I see glamorous women who survived treatment, I am humbled and grateful to be in their company."

— MARGIT, *age 39, diagnosed 1995*

"Going for a walk each morning and knowing I have another day to enjoy the sunrise makes me happy."

— MAUREEN, *age 54, diagnosed 1998*

"In August, we had a very special family get-together at the Connecticut shore. Among the aunts, uncles, cousins, and siblings gathered were several of us who had survived cancer. It was the first time we had all been together at the same time, in the same place. Besides myself, there were two of my sisters and an aunt who have all had breast cancer. There was a cousin who went through a grueling year of treatment for leukemia, and another cousin who'd had breast cancer in 1990 had just finished treatment for ovarian cancer four weeks before. It was an amazing, high-energy day, filled with laughter, story sharing, and picture taking. My cousin who had battled both breast and ovarian cancer summed it up as she looked around at all of us with a huge grin and said, 'We're survivors. We will write a new chapter for this family.'"

— SUSAN, *age 57, diagnosed 1996*

"I have been fortunate to have been a witness to people close to me that have faced life challenges with courage. God has also given me hurdles to cross, but I know there is always a better tomorrow, and when the skies are blue, I fly in them."

— ANITA, *age 59, diagnosed 1991*

"During chemo, I was worried about missing out on my children's lives. Now I am expecting my third child. Joy for me is being alive and providing happiness for my husband and children."

— KRISTINE, *age 33, diagnosed 1998*

"Seven months after I completed my treatment, I took a trip to the Galápagos Islands. Living on a boat on the equator for two weeks definitely helped me to feel 'centered,' but the real joy came from surrounding myself with thousands of healthy boobies (blue-footed, masked, and red-footed varieties)."

— MARGIT, *age 39, diagnosed 1995*

"Six days after I took the final Cytoxan pills, my family and I brought home a puppy. As I watched him in my daughter's arms, I wondered which one of us would survive the other. I hoped he would be a comfort to her if I died. He is now ninety pounds of healthy creature, and I love him beyond all proper proportions for a dog. He is my commitment to a future and represents my hope."

— HESTER, *age 50, diagnosed 1993*

"What makes me happy? Well, that's an easy one— clean pathology reports, clean mammograms, good blood reports, and the days of the year I don't have to think about such things."

— JANA, *age 34, diagnosed 1998*

"What makes me happy? How could I not be happy
with a husband like B.G. (our forty-third wedding
anniversary is tomorrow), with a wonderful family and
soon-to-be-eleven grandchildren, with many many
friends, with gardens to grow, books to read, afghans
to knit, and trips to take. When seven-eighths of the
world's population lives a far less privileged existence,
I can only rejoice in my incredible good fortune."

— RAYA, *age 64, diagnosed 1990*

"My husband and I moved to a small condo after I
finished treatment. The children are off at college, and
we enjoy traveling without having to worry about a big
house. We feel young again. Happy to be alive."

— HOLLY, *age 49, diagnosed 1997*

"Now is the time to look at your life and decide if you are living it the way that you want to. If not, make the changes that you've been wanting to make in order to increase the joy in your life. Even if feeling joyful does not increase the length of your life (though I believe it has the ability to), it will certainly improve your quality of life."

— FRAN, *age 48, diagnosed 1997*

"Birthdays make me happy."

— SONIA, *age 32, diagnosed 1999*

"I love to entertain. I am happy when friends come over to visit."

— ROBIN, *age 38, diagnosed 1996, 1998 & 1999*

"What makes me happy? Well, for a long time after treatment, it was antidepressants. Now what makes me happy is distance from treatment. Not thinking about the past or the future too much. Living now."

— MARY, *age 45, diagnosed 1995 & 1998*

"This may be superficial, but I get great joy from brushing my hair. I missed it when it was gone. Now I French braid it, put clips and ribbons in it, and buy all sorts of pretty barrettes to show it off. I'll never complain about having a bad hair day again!"

— FAITH, *age 41, diagnosed 1997*

"Each spring, I buy tickets to the Stars on Ice tour to see Scott Hamilton skate. His energy and ability to return to his art seemingly unscathed after his bout with cancer are totally inspiring. He's unstoppable! He's funny, poetic, and graceful. Watching him always puts a smile on my face. The man had chemo, and he still does back flips!"

— MARGIT, *age 39, diagnosed 1995*

"Breast cancer was my wake-up call. It scared the heck out of me, but surviving treatment made me feel stronger. I work at taking care of myself now, finding joy (something I never used to do). I go to bed earlier, eat better, and don't waste time with negative people."

— DAWN, *age 48, diagnosed 1999*

"Three days after I was diagnosed with breast cancer, my boyfriend of five years proposed to me and moved from Florida to take care of me during treatment. I quit work and focused on planning my wedding. The entire time I was going through treatment, I had my wedding to look forward to. Even though I got really sick from chemo, I was happy because I kept thinking about marrying this wonderful man. I'm now happily, healthily married. My favorite times are holidays—spending time with my husband doing anything and nothing."

— TIFANY, *age 25, diagnosed 1996*

"I love spending time with my grandchildren."

— SUSAN, *age 58, diagnosed 1997*

"A dear friend and I (diagnosed two years apart) have great fun with THE WIZARD OF OZ theme. It began with admiring a fun pair of ruby slipper earrings she'd been sent. Later I gave her a doll-size ruby glitter slipper. I started using Oz-related cards with gifts. She made me a cassette tape of 'Over the Rainbow' renditions and even gave me an Oz banner just before my chest wall resection. The little gifts we trade have multiple symbolism: our path or journey with friends, facing fear and finding bravery, wondering what's over the rainbow, and always the safety of home by clicking those ruby slippers. As we travel on a sometimes parallel path, our Oz preoccupation stretches across the abyss of blackness and connects light to light."

— CINDY, *age 47, diagnosed 1993 & 1997*

"All of my training for Mount Fuji is done between 5:20 and 6:30-ish A.M. Without my 'Fuji focus,' there's no way I would be able to be walking into a gym at 5:18 in the morning! I began this program on Martin Luther King Day, which was very symbolic for me, since treatment ended one year before, almost to the day. I thought it would be difficult to get going, especially getting up in the cold and pitch-dark, and then going outside on some mornings in eight-degree temperatures and/or with snow and ice on the ground. Surprisingly, though, I NEVER feel cold. I only feel focused and determined.

"As spring is coming to New Jersey, there is an inspiring and immediate reward at the end of the workout. All this week, I have been greeted with the

❧

most amazing sunrises as I walk out of the gym. I've had to stop in my sweaty tracks just to watch, and all I can think about is how wonderful it is to be alive, to feel as if I'm in control again, and how amazing it will be to watch the sun rise over Fuji!"

— *Team Member, Climb Against the Odds—Mount Fuji 2000,*
LINDA RINALDI, *age 46, diagnosed 1998*

Resources

Contacts for helpful information,

comfort, and fun.

N E W S   F L A S H !

"HOT FLASHES, A DREADED SIDE EFFECT of menopause, have many of us talking about how to rid ourselves of the nasty problem. From personal experience, I can tell you that relaxing through the hormonal change is one great step in the right direction. Yes, hot flashes are awful! There is no arguing that. But so are menstrual cramps and water retention. Sometimes the least complicated solutions are the best.

"Just after my thirty-eighth birthday, I was thrown into surgical menopause. The instant lack of hormones presented the usual set of problems, but I was determined not to let them get the better of me. In general, I found that exercise, yoga, and eating more soy and fewer carbohydrates seemed to help a bit. A good attitude helped, too. But let's face it, when you're wearing a beautiful silk blouse and your body does this flash flood thing, it's pretty hard to stay peppy and positive.

"It was at the annual Northeast Coop organic food fair that I discovered the solution to my hot flashes. I was dressed in layers so that I could keep taking off and putting on clothes as the need arose. Finally, when even my bra was soaked, I began to feel sorry for myself. I walked up to one of the booths that was selling herbs and homeopathic remedies and asked, 'Do you have anything for menopausal symptoms?' A woman handed me valerian and kava for sleep, a moisturizer for my skin, and a lubricant for sex. 'What about hot flashes? If one can't take hormones, what do you offer for relieving hot flashes?' I asked. The woman smiled and handed me a hand-held Japanese fan. I laughed, but guess what? It works!"

— MARGIT, *age 39, diagnosed 1995*

YOGA POSTURES & DESCRIPTIONS

*(Consult with your health care professional about the risks
and benefits of yoga before trying these exercises.)*

VIPARITA KARANI
"Topsy-Turvy Pose"

The Topsy-Turvy Pose
reverses the pull of gravity
on your legs, creates a soft
back bend in the trunk,
opens the lungs and heart,
and eases nausea and anxiety.

Directions

Lie on your back with your
hips resting on a bolster and a
blanket and pillow supporting
your head. Place your legs
up against the wall. Cover
your eyes with a rice bag.

SAVASANA VARIATION
"Relaxation Pose"

This pose promotes full, deep relaxation. It gives the sensation that your body is floating and leaves you with a warm, safe feeling.

Directions

Lie on your back with a bolster supporting your chest, a blanket supporting your shoulders and head, a roll under your neck, a roll under your knees, and pillows supporting your arms. Place a rice bag over your eyes.

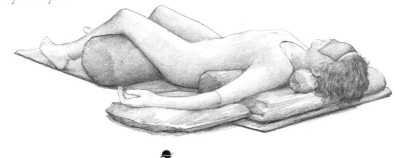

Illustrations by Erick Ingraham

GHARBASANA
"Supported Child's Pose"

This is a passive, supported forward bend. It's good for easing lower back discomfort and is very restful.

Directions

Starting from a kneeling position, bend your knees and rest your hips on your heels. Place a bolster between your knees and rest your chest and head on the bolster. Support both arms with pillows.

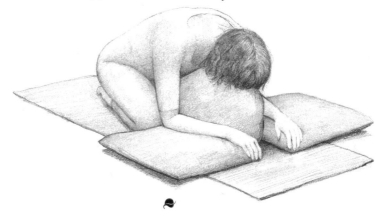

SIDE-LYING POSE

The Side-Lying Pose creates a soft twist in
your body and releases your lower back.

Directions

Lying on the floor, turn your body so that
your chest and head are supported by a pillow
and your head is also resting on a blanket.

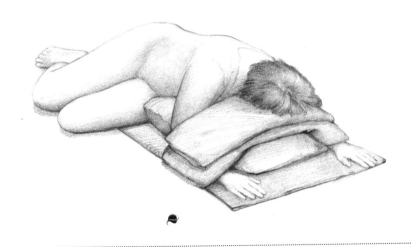

UPAVISTHA KONASANA VARIATION
"Wide-Angle Pose with Chair"

Forward bends like this and the next one
quiet the mind, release tension headaches,
gently open the back, and relax the heart.

Directions

Place a chair in front of you, then sit on
the floor. Rest your head and arms on the
·chair, supporting them with a blanket.

UPAVISTHA KONASANA VARIATION
"Wide-Angle Pose with Bolster"

Directions

Sitting on the floor, pull a
bolster in close, so it places
a gentle pressure on your
belly. Place a blanket on
top of the bolster and rest
your head and arms on
the blanket and bolster.

SETU BANDHA
"Supported-Bridge Pose with Arms at Side"

This position and the next one open the chest and promote deep breathing.

Directions

Lie on your back with your hips resting on a bolster, your shoulders resting on a blanket, your head supported by a roll, and your arms out to the side.

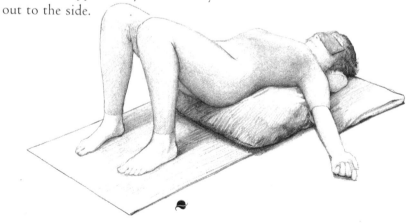

SETU BANDHA
"Supported-Bridge Pose with Arms Up"

Directions

Lying on your back, rest
your hips on a bolster and
your shoulders and head on a
pillow. Stretch your arms up
over your head.

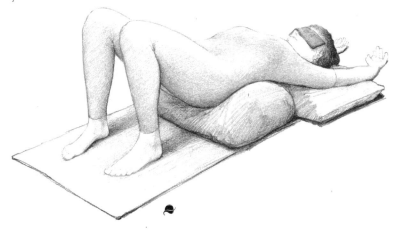

Yoga postures and descriptions provided by Carol Nelson, Creative Yoga Studio, Brookline, Massachusetts

BREAST CANCER–RELATED ORGANIZATIONS

IF YOU HAVE BEEN THINKING ABOUT fighting breast cancer on a level bigger than the cells in your body, here are just a few organizations that will help you get moving. Some sponsor walks and races or help shape public policy. Others offer opportunities to go fishing, rafting, or mountain climbing, or just help you get back on your feet. But all of these breast cancer organizations raise awareness and funds with one common goal—eradicating breast cancer. These listings are for national headquarters. Start with them to identify resources available in your area.

American Cancer Society

1599 Clifton Road NE, Atlanta, GA 30329

800-ACS-2345   877-333-HOPE   www.cancer.org

Programs include Cancer Survivors Network, Reach to Recovery, Look Good—Feel Better, Adventure Weekend, Making Strides Against Breast Cancer, and Relay for Life, as well as many other informative and educational services and events.

American Institute for Cancer Research

1759 R Street NW, Washington, DC 20009

800-843-8114   202-328-7744   www.aicr.org

Education and research programs include the AICR NEWS-LETTER, AICR Health Aids, Cancer Resource, AICR Education Seminars, and Pen Pals Network.

American Menopause Foundation Inc.

350 Fifth Avenue, Suite 2822, New York, NY 10118

212-714-2398   www.americanmenopause.org

Support and assistance on all issues concerning menopause. Through a newsletter, other literature, and educational programs, it provides the latest information on scientific research and other pertinent facts regarding menopause.

The Anderson Network

1515 Holcombe Boulevard, Box 216, Houston, TX 77030

800-345-6324   713-792-2553

http:/www.mdacc.tmc.edu/centers/pathway/andnet/index.html

This organization connects you with an Anderson Network member (current or former patient of the M. D. Anderson Cancer Center) with a diagnosis and treatment like yours.

Breast Cancer Action

55 New Montgomery Street, Suite 323, San Francisco, CA 94105

877-2STOPBC   415-243-9301   www.bcaction.org

Breast Cancer Action carries the voices of people affected by breast cancer to inspire and compel the changes necessary to end the breast cancer epidemic. Founded and led by women living with breast cancer, the organization offers programs that provide information, give people something to do (besides worry about breast cancer), and advocate for policy changes that will lead to true prevention, a real cure, and universal access to quality care.

The Breast Cancer Fund

2107 O'Farrell Street @Divisadero, San Francisco, CA 94115-3419

866-760-TBCF   415-346-TBCF   www.breastcancerfund.org

Its mission is to end breast cancer through research, action, and policy initiatives that support (1) replacement of mammography with safer, more reliable detection methods; (2) nontoxic treatments; (3) elimination of preventable causes of the disease, including those in the environment; and (4) access to the best available medical care and information for everyone. The Fund creates awareness and funding through mountain climbs and physical challenges; art exhibits; films; and cutting-edge advocacy campaigns, conferences, and educational materials. Copies of the videotapes CLIMB AGAINST THE ODDS and BREAST CANCER AND RECOVERY are available for purchase through the Fund.

Cancer Care Inc.

275 Seventh Avenue, New York, NY 10001

800-813-HOPE   212-302-2400   www.cancercare.org

Support, information, and practical help for people with cancer and their loved ones. Services are provided by oncology social workers and are available in person, over the telephone, and through the agency's Web site. Cancer Care's reach also extends to professionals, providing education, information, and assistance. All services are offered at no charge.

Casting for Recovery

PMB-257, 946 Great Plain Avenue, Needham, MA 02492-3030

888-553-3500   CFRProgram@aol.com

This group offers weekend fly-fishing instruction in a beautiful setting, along with group discussions, networking, and time to connect with the natural world. Lodging and food are included. Retreats are held across the country and are free to all participants.

Healthtalk Interactive

201 Queen Anne Avenue North, Seattle, WA 98109

800-672-4677   206-233-0135   www.healthtalk.com

This Seattle-based organization is devoted to providing the latest information and support to people coping with many serious conditions, including breast cancer.

The Susan G. Komen Breast Cancer Foundation

5005 LBJ Freeway, Suite 250, Dallas, TX 75244

800-I'M AWARE   972-855-1600   www.breastcancerinfo.com

The Komen Foundation is fighting to eradicate breast cancer as a life-threatening disease by advancing research, education, screening, and treatment. Proceeds from the Foundation's Komen Race for the Cure — a series of 5k runs/fitness walks—fund national and international research efforts and local breast health and breast outreach programs.

Living Beyond Breast Cancer

10 East Athens Avenue, Suite 204, Admore, PA 19003

888-753-5222   610-645-4567   www.lbbc.org

Dedicated to empowering all women affected by breast cancer to live as long as possible with the best possible quality of life. Programs include a newsletter, conferences, community outreach programs, a help line, and a networking group.

The Men's Crusade Against Breast Cancer

4502 Fidelity Court, Annandale, VA 22003

703-978-3336

Dedicated to mobilizing men and families in the war on breast cancer and raising awareness that it is a family issue.

The National Alliance
of Breast Cancer Organizations

9 East Thirty-seventh Street, New York, NY 10016

888-80-NABCO   212-889-0606   www.nabco.org

The Avon Breast Cancer 3-DAY is an outdoor sixty-mile awareness and fundraising walk taking place in several cities. The net proceeds raised by the Avon Breast Cancer 3-DAY are awarded as grants through the Avon Breast Cancer Awareness Crusade to community-based programs that link medically underserved women to breast cancer education and screening services. NABCO, Avon's national program partner in administering the grants, is a network of breast cancer organizations that provides assistance and information to anyone with questions about breast cancer. All of NABCO's services are free to the public.

The National Breast Cancer Coalition

1701 L Street NW, Suite 1060, Washington, DC 20036

800-622-2838   202-296-7477   www.stopbreastcancer.org

A grassroots network of more than five hundred member organizations and sixty thousand individual members, NBCC is a catalyst that moves our country toward greater awareness of breast cancer and more effective strategies to eradicate this deadly disease. NBCC educates its members, enabling them to become partners with scientists to design research and help determine how federal breast cancer research funds are spent. Through its many programs, NBCC continues to develop strategies to improve access to quality health care for all women and to train its constituency to deliver accurate, informed, and up-to-date information about breast cancer to the public and policymakers.

National Cancer Institute

31 Center Drive, Bethesda, MD 20892

800-4-CANCER 301-496-5583 http://www.nci.nih.gov

Provides the latest cancer information to patients and their families, as well as to the public and health professionals.

National Cancer Survivors Day Foundation

P.O. Box 682285, Franklin, TN 37068-2285

615-794-3006 www.ncsdf.org

The National Cancer Survivors Day Foundation sponsors North America's annual celebration of life for cancer survivors and their families, friends, and oncology teams. The celebration takes place each year on the first Sunday in June.

National Coalition for Cancer Survivorship

1010 Wayne Avenue, Silver Spring, MD 20910

877-NCCS-YES   301-650-9127   www.cancersearch.org

Unites all those touched by cancer. Programs such as Rays of Hope, Ribbon of Hope, and The March deal with many issues concerning cancer survivorship.

National Lymphedema Network

2211 Post Street, Suite 404, San Francisco, CA 94115-3427

800-541-3259   415-921-1306   www.lymphnet.org

Provides information, education, referrals, and support regarding lymphedema. Services include a newsletter, resource guide, and lymphedema alert jewelry.

Northeast Health Care Quality Foundation

15 Old Rollinsford Road, Suite 302, Dover, NH 03820-2830

603-749-1641

Conceived and implements the Bells and Silence for Remembrance and It's My Fight Too campaigns, which honor those who have been touched by breast cancer and encourage families to be supported as well.

Patient Advocate Foundation

780 Pilot House Drive, Suite 100-C, Newport News, VA 23606

800-532-5274   757-873-6668   www.patientadvocate.org

This network for health care reform provides patient rights information relative to health insurance and legal issues.

Silent Spring Institute

29 Crafts Street, Newton, MA 02458

617-332-4288   www.silentspring.org

Silent Spring builds on a unique partnership of scientists,
physicians, public health advocates, and community activists
who are dedicated to identifying and breaking the links
between the environment and breast cancer. The institute
is committed to breast cancer prevention, a research agenda
with an activist vision that goes far beyond science as usual.

The Wellness Community

2716 Ocean Park Boulevard, Suite 1040, Santa Monica, CA 90405
888-793-WELL   310-314-2555

Provides ongoing and drop-in support groups facilitated by licensed psychotherapists; body work such as yoga and tai chi; relaxation, visualization, and meditation; a writing program; educational workshops in areas such as nutrition; and an "Ask the Doctor" series. Parties, joke fests, and get-togethers are part of The Wellness Community's programs.

World Conference on Breast Cancer

841 Princess Street, Kingston, Ontario K7L1G7 Canada

613-549-1118   www.brcancerconf.kos.net

This is an international conference at which experts from around the world gather and share their knowledge and information about breast cancer.

MAIL-ORDER PRODUCTS

Aubrey Organics

4419 North Manhattan Avenue, Tampa, FL 33614

800-AUBREY-H   813-876-8166   www.aubrey-organics.com

Hair and skin products that do not contain synthetic chemicals and use all-natural and many organic ingredients.

L.A. Burdick

Main Street, P.O. Box 593, Walpole, NH 03608

800-229-2419   603-756-3701   www.burdickchocolate.com

When it comes to fine chocolate, it doesn't get any better than this!

Enhancement Inc.

P.O. Box 867, Morro Bay, CA 93443-0867

888-584-9633   805-771-8640   www.enhancementinc.com

Offers a video—FOCUS ON HEALING THROUGH MOVEMENT & DANCE FOR THE BREAST CANCER SURVIVOR—of a dance-based exercise routine for survivors to use at home.

Healing Adventures

5323 Rosalind Avenue, Richmond, CA 94805

510-237-8291   boatfun@igc.org   www.wenet.net/-stcohan

Provides a range of healing adventures in nature for those recovering from illness, as well as their family and friends.

Living Arts

P.O. Box 2908, Venice, CA 90291-2908

800-254-8464   www.livingarts.com

Catalog of products for yoga and total well-being, such as clothing, props, and an excellent assortment of instructional self-help videos, books, and music.

MAMM Magazine

349 West Twelfth Street, New York, NY 10014

888-901-MAMM   212-242-2163   www.Mamm.com

A consumer publication devoted to breast and women's reproductive cancers.

Natural Habitat Adventures

11266 West Hillsborough Avenue, Suite 344, Tampa, FL 33635

877-4-NATHAB   813-282-9011   www.nathab.com

Specializes in customizing "soft" adventure vacations for small groups of twelve to fourteen people. Not an "ing" company. That is, it is not about hiking, biking, and bungee jumping.

Nutrition Action Healthletter

1875 Connecticut Avenue NW, Suite 300, Washington, DC 20009

202-332-9110   www.cspinet.org

A newsletter about nutrition and food, published by the Center for Science in the Public Interest.

The Original Bug Shirt

Box 127, Trout Creek, Ontario, P0H2L0 Canada

800-998-9096 705-729-5620 www.bugshirt.com

Nothing about this shirt will bug you! It's great for protecting yourself from bug bites and sun.

Solarcare Pharmaceutical Inc.

1015-A Main Street, Evansville, IN 47708-1824

800-489-4453 812-421-4454 solarcare@netzero.net

Sun care products that are natural and chemical-free, with ingredients derived from organic and renewable resources.

E. Shan Tang

157 Harvard Avenue, Allston, MA 02134

617-787-4503   EShanTang@aol.com

Provides Chinese herbs and information on wellness.

Tempur-Pedic

1713 Jaggie Fox Way, Lexington, KY 40511

800-814-1268   606-259-0754   www.tempurpedic.com

The Tempur-Pedic Swedish Sleep System automatically
reacts to your body's weight, shape, and temperature, giving
you a sense of weightlessness that promotes a deep sleep.
Great for postoperative comfort.

Yoga Props

3055 Twenty-third Street, San Francisco, CA 94110
888-856-YOGA   415-285-YOGA   yogaprops@sfo.com

Ask for its catalog of great yoga stuff. Offers many videos and books; an excellent source for bolsters, benches, and ropes.

Yoga Zone

3342 Melrose Avenue NW, Roanoke, VA 24017
888-264-9642   www.yogazone.com

Yoga products for yuppies—jewelry, clothing, and really nice sticky mats, bolsters, and eye pillows. Ask for a catalog.

If the Order Form Is Missing...

...AND YOU WOULD LIKE TO OBTAIN COPIES OF HOPE LIVES! please write on a piece of paper your name, address, phone number, and the number of books you would like, and send it to us with your payment of $13.50 per book (includes shipping and handling).

We enjoy hearing from you, so feel free just to drop us a line with your comments and tell us how you heard about HOPE LIVES!

HOPE LIVES!
P.O. Box 3026
Peterborough, N.H. 03458

Order Form

TO OBTAIN COPIES OF HOPE LIVES! please fill out this order form and mail it to us with your payment of $13.50 (includes shipping and handling) per book. If you do not wish to tear out this page or you need more space for comments, please feel free to write the information on a separate piece of paper.

1. Name: . . . .

2. Address and phone number: . . . .

. . . .

3. How did you hear about this book? . . . .

. . . .

HOPE LIVES! P.O. Box 3026, Peterborough, N.H. 03458

Acknowledgments

THE FOLLOWING PEOPLE AND CORPORATIONS not only helped make this book possible but made publishing it a pleasurable experience. I and this small book have been blessed with the help of so many people. Thank you to all of you who created HOPE LIVES! and who keep hope alive!

Dr. Margaret Duggan, Dr. Annette Furst, Dr. Ronald Garrell, Dr. Linda Lauretti, Dr. Kathleen Mayzel, Anne McManus, Janet Rustow, Dr. Norman Sadowsky, Dr. Alan Semine, Dr. Benjamin Smith, and the entire staff at the Faulkner Hospital, Boston; Judith Hirshfield Bartek, Dr. Carolyn Lamb, and Elizabeth Stamos of the Beth Israel Deaconess Medical Center, Boston; Dr. Michael Muto and Anne Kelly of Brigham and Women's Hospital and the Dana-Farber Cancer Institute; Blue Cross Blue Shield of New Hampshire; Capital City Press; Eastern Mountain Sports; The

Acknowledgments

Frank Foundation; Genentech Inc.; Granite Bank; Al Melanson Co.; Danielle (Glinda), Barbara, Deborah, Julia, John, and Tina of the Monadnock Community Hospital, Peterborough, New Hampshire; Oxford University Press; The Peterborough Town Library; Quad Graphics; Rosaly's Farmstand (grower and giver of the beautiful lupine on the cover); Stonyfield Farm; Team Fuji 2000; Doreen Abraham; Mr. and Mrs. Ian Alexander; John Baskin; The Bean Family; Steve Berg; Mr. and Mrs. David Brownwood; Fred Bruemmer; Mr. and Mrs. Christopher Cappy; Dr. and Mrs. Gilbert Cogan; Perry Colmore; Dr. Jorge Crespo; Jim Crowley; Andrew Davis, Esq.; Mr. and Mrs. William Doeren; Clark Dumont; Heather Fletcher; Daniel Gonsalves; Mr. and Mrs. Alex Gould; Josie Gould; Mr. and Mrs. Neil Halliday; Mr. and Mrs. Mike Harde; Marcie Hawley; Mr. and Mrs. Hiroshi Hayashi; Mr. and Mrs. Roy Hayward; Barbara Huebner; Erick Ingraham; Mr. and Mrs. Karl Jacobsen; Barbara Jatkola; Mr. and Mrs. Court Johnson; Nikala Johnson; Mr. and

Mrs. Tom Judd; Mr. and Mrs. Robert Kaufmann; Nat Lawton; Mr. and Mrs. Charles Letovsky; Mr. and Mrs. Norman Makechnie; Dr. Michael Maki; Andrea R. Martin; Mr. and Mrs. Reagan Messer; Doug Mindell; Lucy Miskin; Mr. and Mrs. William Mitchell; Richard Nash; Naya; Carol Nelson; Barbara Pastan; Mr. and Mrs. Andrew Peterson; Mr. and Mrs. Edward Petrilli; Cynthia Porter; J Porter; Mr. and Mrs. Clifford Potter; Dr. Robert Provost; Mr. and Mrs. Robert Ray; Evelyn Rhodes; Karen Rouse; Jack Russell; Dr. and Mrs. David Serra; Claudette Silver; Mr. and Mrs. Stephen Siwek; Marianne Shaughnessy; Kathy Smith; my editor, Sharon Smith; Margaret A. Storer Jr.; Mr. and Mrs. Glen Swanson; Kent Swig; Greg Tobin (MAJOR BIG THANKS!); Terry Vose and Judi (soon to be Mrs.); B. J. Wang; Mr. and Mrs. Peter Ward; Mr. and Mrs. Peter White; Mr. and Mrs. Jay Worthen; Dave Ziarnowski; and once again the town of Peterborough, New Hampshire, as well as the hundreds of women across the country who authored this book.

❧

"But the symbols of hope

are not lacking even in the grayness and bleakness of the winter sea. On land we know that the apparent lifelessness of winter is an illusion. Look closely at the bare branches of a tree, on which not the palest gleam of green can be discerned. Yet, spaced along each branch are the leaf buds, all the spring's magic of swelling green concealed and safely preserved under the insulating, overlapping layers. Pick off a piece of the rough bark of the trunk; there you will find hibernating insects. Dig down through the snow into the earth. There are the eggs of next summer's grasshoppers; there are the dormant seeds from which will come the grass, the herb, the oak tree."

—RACHEL CARSON, *The Sea Around Us*

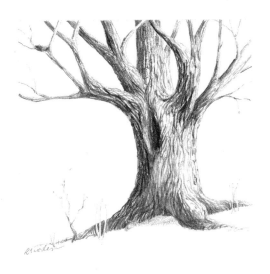

— WINTER LANDSCAPE, *pencil by Evelyn Rhodes, age 53, diagnosed 1990*